WHEN HOPE CHANGES

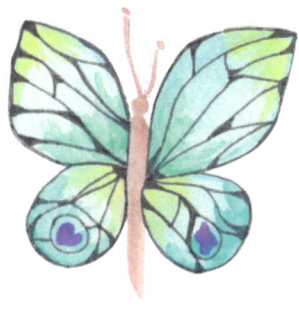

ISBN 979-8-218-32206-9

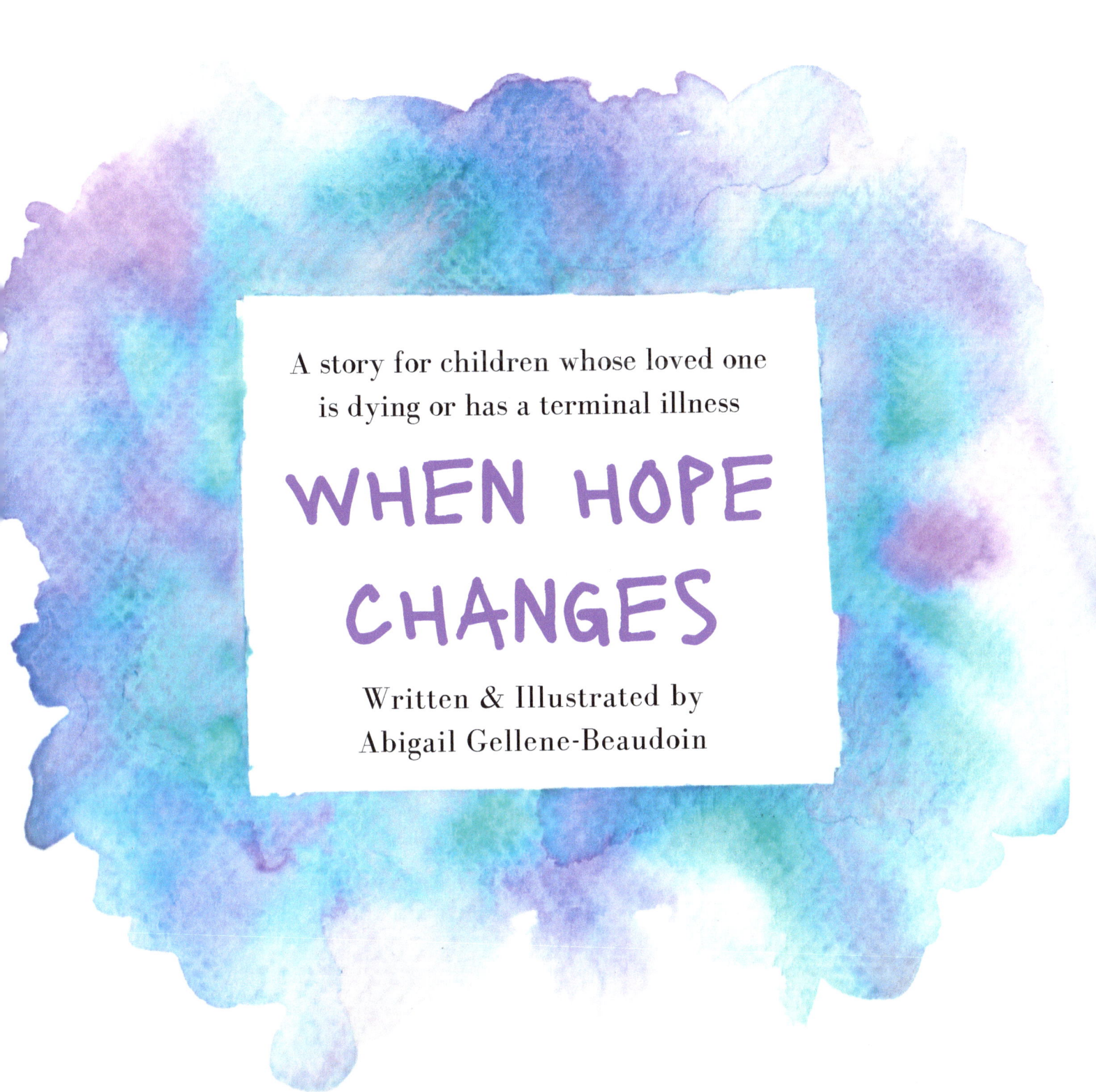

A story for children whose loved one
is dying or has a terminal illness

WHEN HOPE CHANGES

Written & Illustrated by
Abigail Gellene-Beaudoin

HOW TO USE THIS BOOK

To the grown-up who plans to use this book to support a child navigating a loved one's end-stage disease or terminal diagnosis: thank you. In doing your best to explain your or your loved one's situation, you are arming your child with knowledge, trust, and permission to feel. Your honesty is a priceless gift.

There are blanks in this book which are intended to be filled with the words or names that fit your situation best. Below each blank is some guidance, but these are intended to be used by you and your family however you deem most appropriate.

In the back of the book, I have compiled some further guidance in terms of sharing medical information. Please use this as you see fit. It may be that your medical team can provide more details or assistance in explaining the diagnosis. Never be afraid to ask for help from your team.

Though this is a non-religious book, some families use their faith and belief background to provide explanation or comfort when facing uncertainty. If that sounds like something that would fit your family, don't hesitate to make margin notes or add in any elements that would meet this need.

Lastly, as you, the loving grown-up, also maneuver the challenges, emotions, and grief that often accompanies an end-stage disease or terminal diagnosis, I urge you to give yourself grace. This is hard and you are doing the best you can.

Dedicated with warm affection to my patients and their families: your indefatigable courage, resilience, and joie de vivre inspire me daily.

Our person, _____, is truly one of a kind.

daddy, grandma, name

There are SO many things we love and admire about them,

and some of my favorites are:_____

_____

_____

_____

_____

their bravery, sense of humor, loving heart, goofy smile etc.

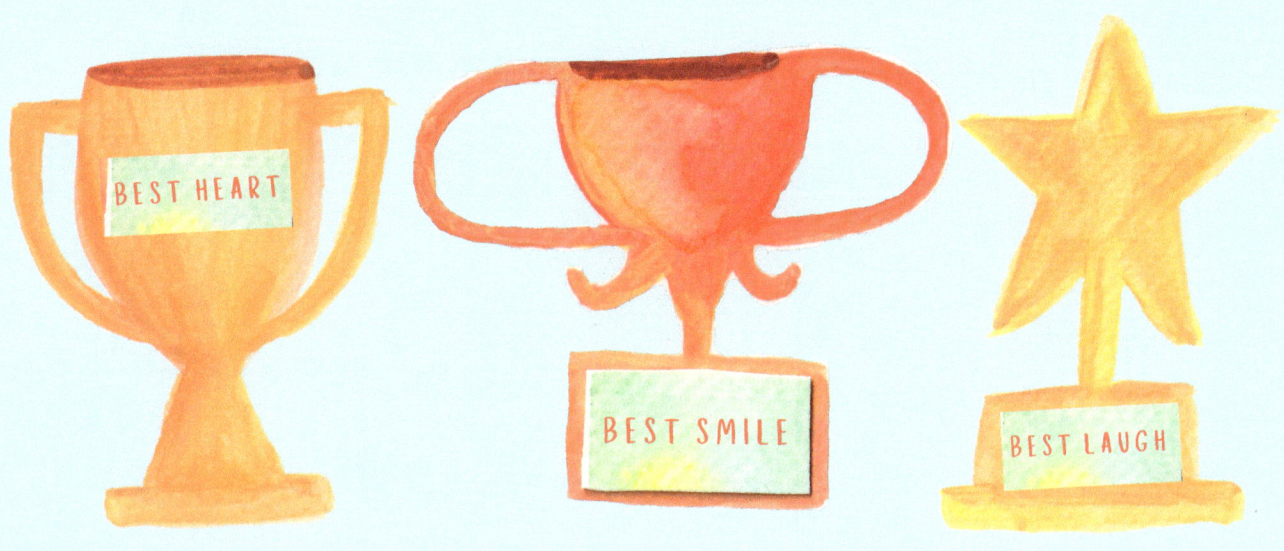

As you may know, our person's body has been very sick. This is because

they have _____, and now their

_____ is having trouble working

like it is supposed to.

This is a problem because _____

_____

_____

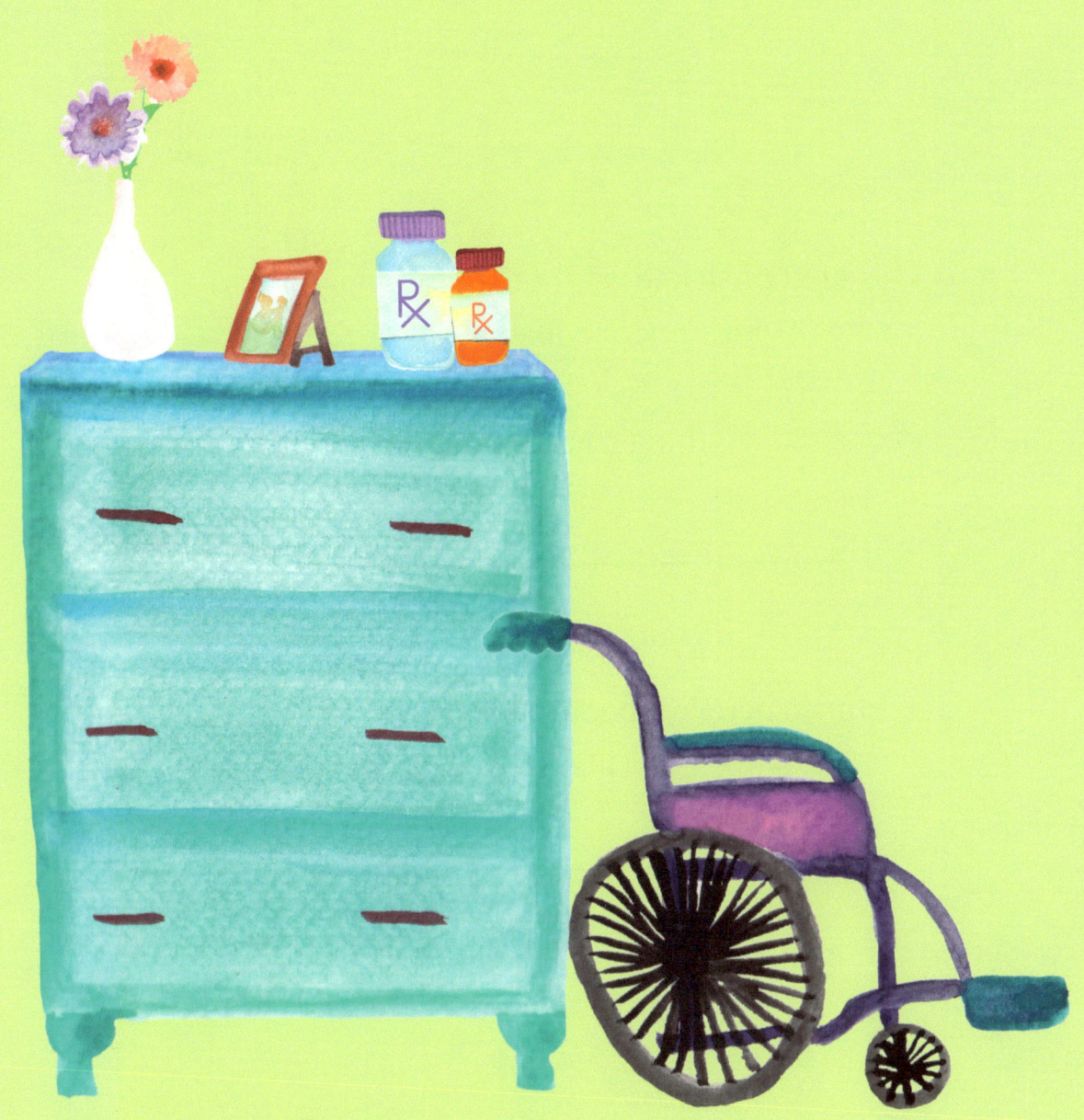

This kind of sickness is not something you can catch from someone like a cold or the flu.

No one did anything to cause our person to have

_____

diagnosis

Sometimes people's bodies just get really sick and don't work like they should.

This is hard for all of us to understand.

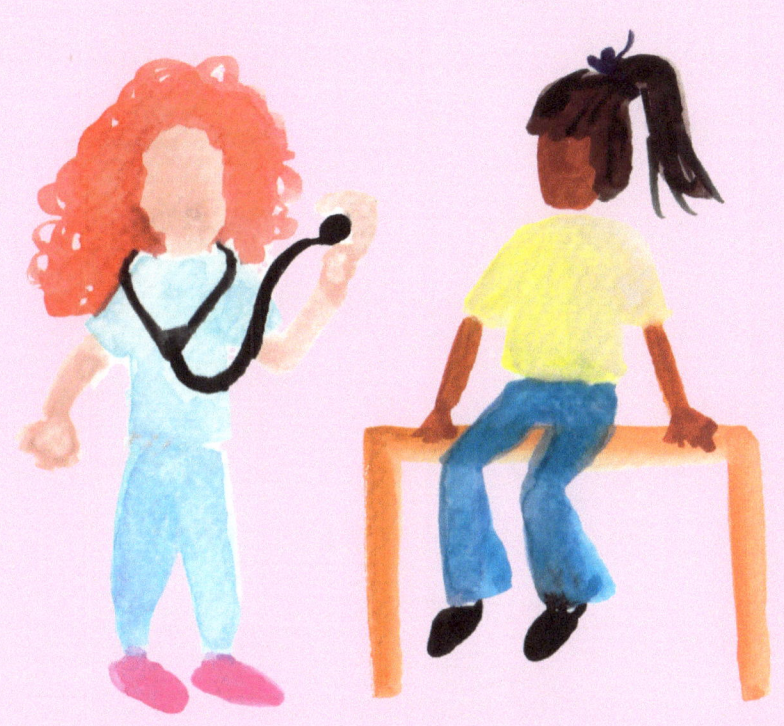

Medicine or surgery can sometimes help when
people's bodies have _____.
diagnosis

Our person's doctors have been hopeful that medicine
can help fix their body.

But recently, the doctors told us that even though they
tried and hoped for our person's body to get better,
the medicine is not working.

This means that our person's body cannot get better
and will not be able to work like it should.

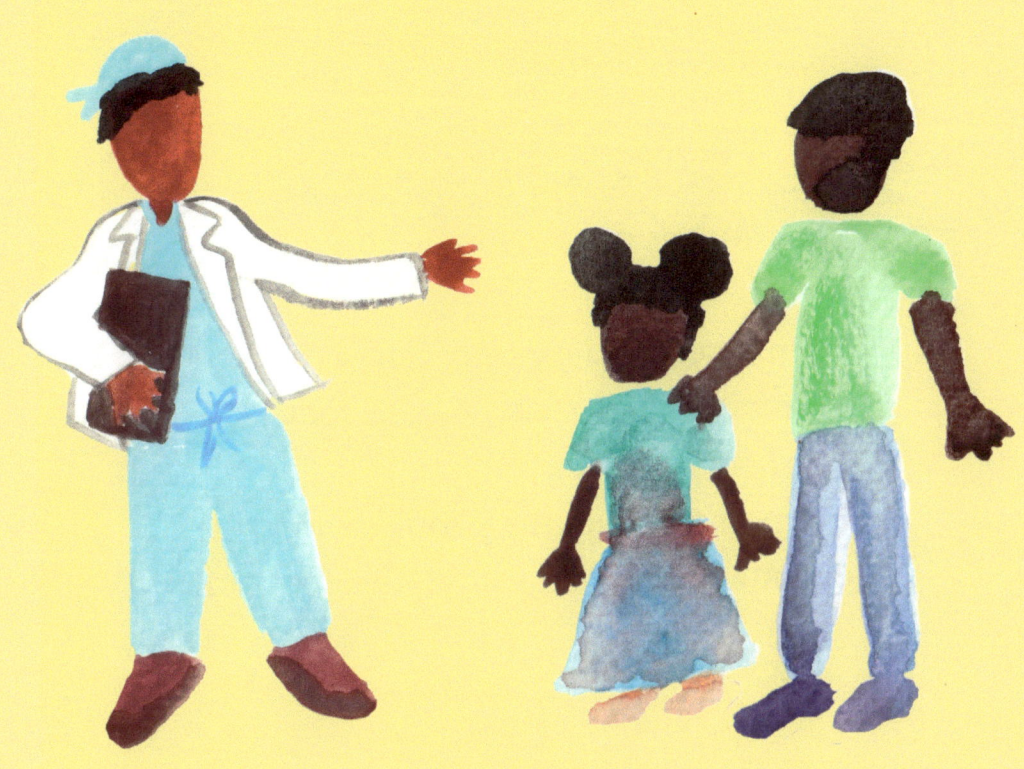

If our person's body doesn't work, that
means our person will die.

When a person dies, they can't breathe,
move, see, touch, hear, or feel.

When people die, the people who love
them miss them and sometimes feel sad.

Thinking about _____ dying makes me makes me feel mad

daddy, grandma, name

Sad

Disappointed

Confused

Impatient

Nervous

Frustrated

Scared

Lonely

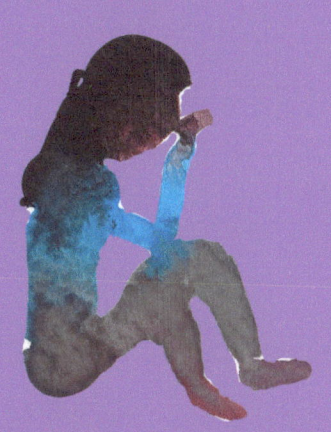

It's okay to feel any of these feelings and more!

Your big feelings are okay, and you don't have to feel them alone. I am with you. We are a team.

When you feel mad, sad, confused, nervous, or any other feeling; you can always come to me for a hug, snuggle, or chat.

It's also okay if there are times you want to be alone. Even in these times, remember I am here for you.

Ask me ANY questions you have, and if I don't know the answer, we will make a list together and we can ask the doctor.

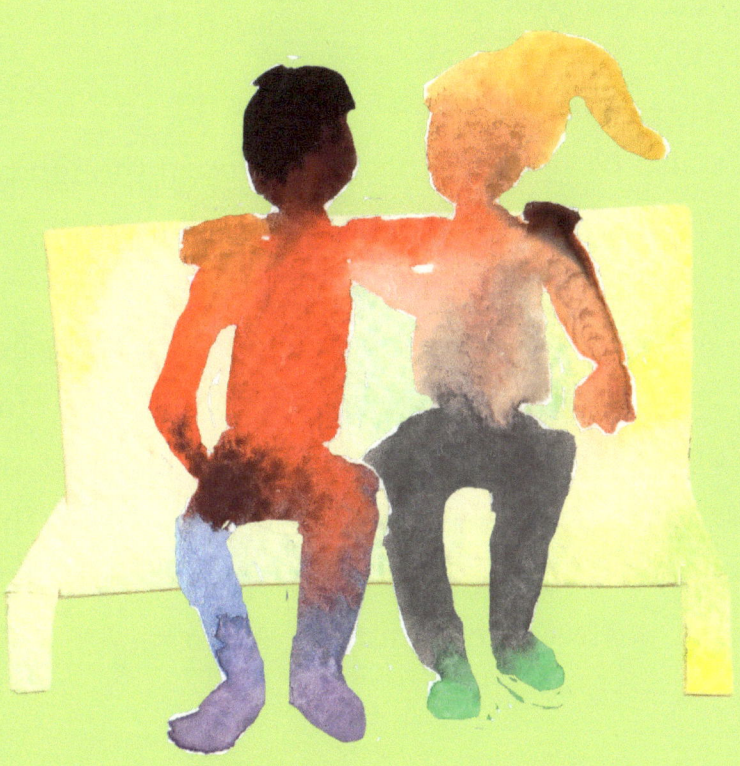

It's also okay to still have hope even though hope may look a little different now.

We were hoping for our person's body to get better, but now we are hoping that they stay comfortable, have as little pain as possible, and are able to feel how much love we have for them.

It sure is a lot of love, isn't it?

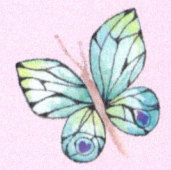
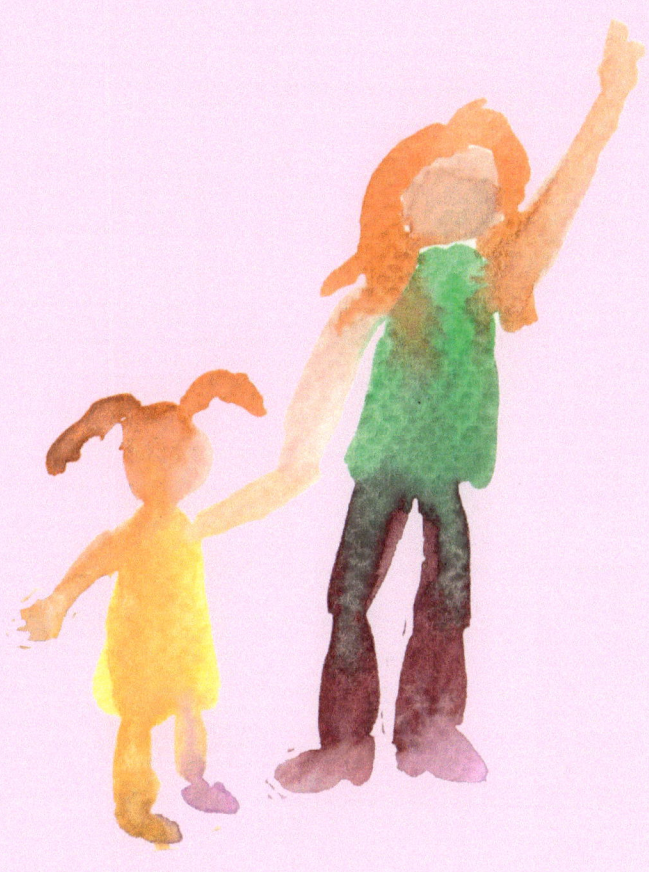

We will tell our person how much we love _____

_____

_____

_____

_____

their bravery, sense of humor, loving heart, goofy smile etc.

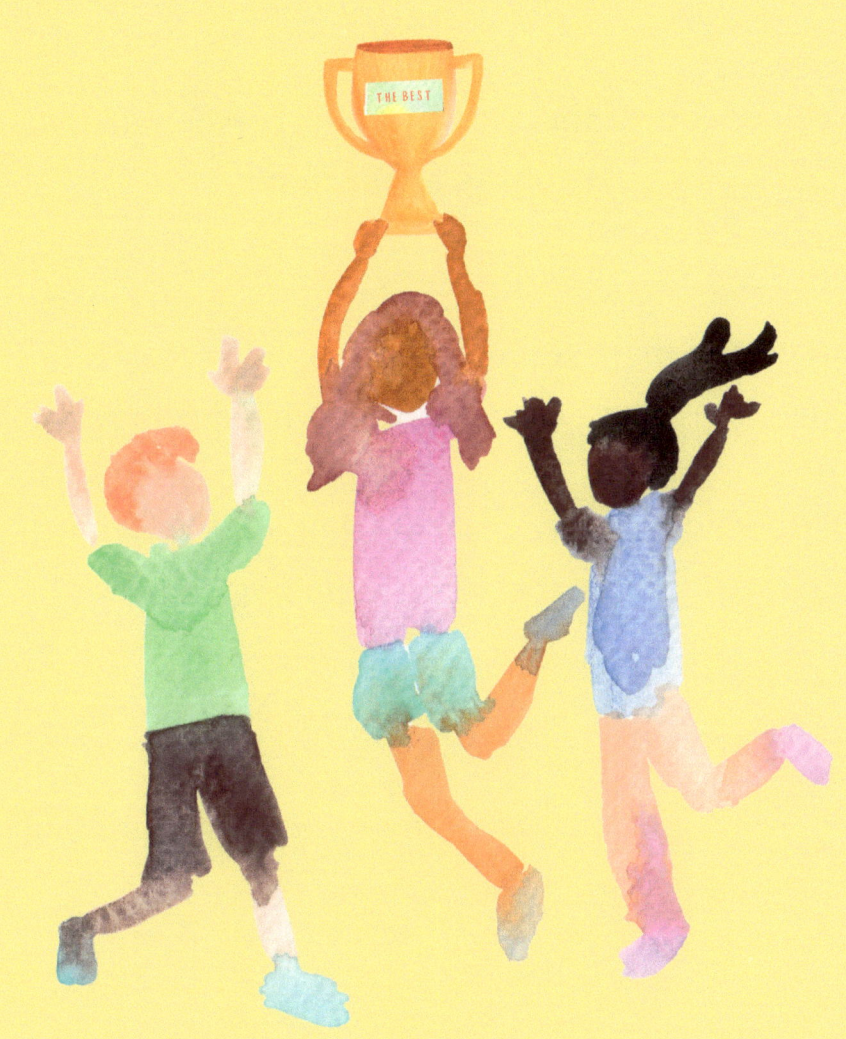

We can do lots of things to help our person feel how much we care about them.

We can talk with them, write them letters, color them pictures, tell them stories, tell them jokes (I'm sure you know some funny ones!), and hold their hand if they want us to!

Our hopes may have changed, but what doesn't change is how special our person is to us.

And also, how special we are to them.

We will always be connected to our person through love.

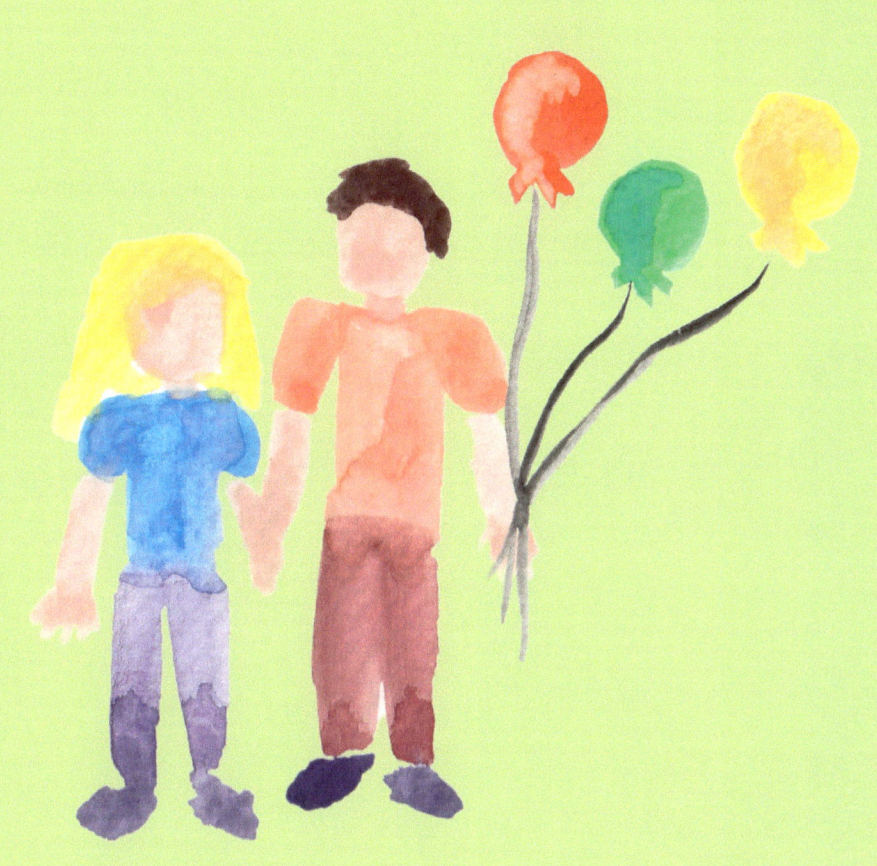

There's no way of knowing for sure how much time we have before our person dies.

I wish there was. Not knowing is hard.

What I do know, is that I will be there for you no matter what, and you are safe to share how you feel.

We can do hard things together.

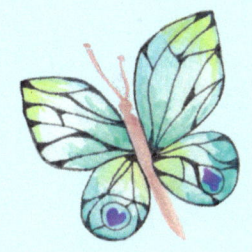

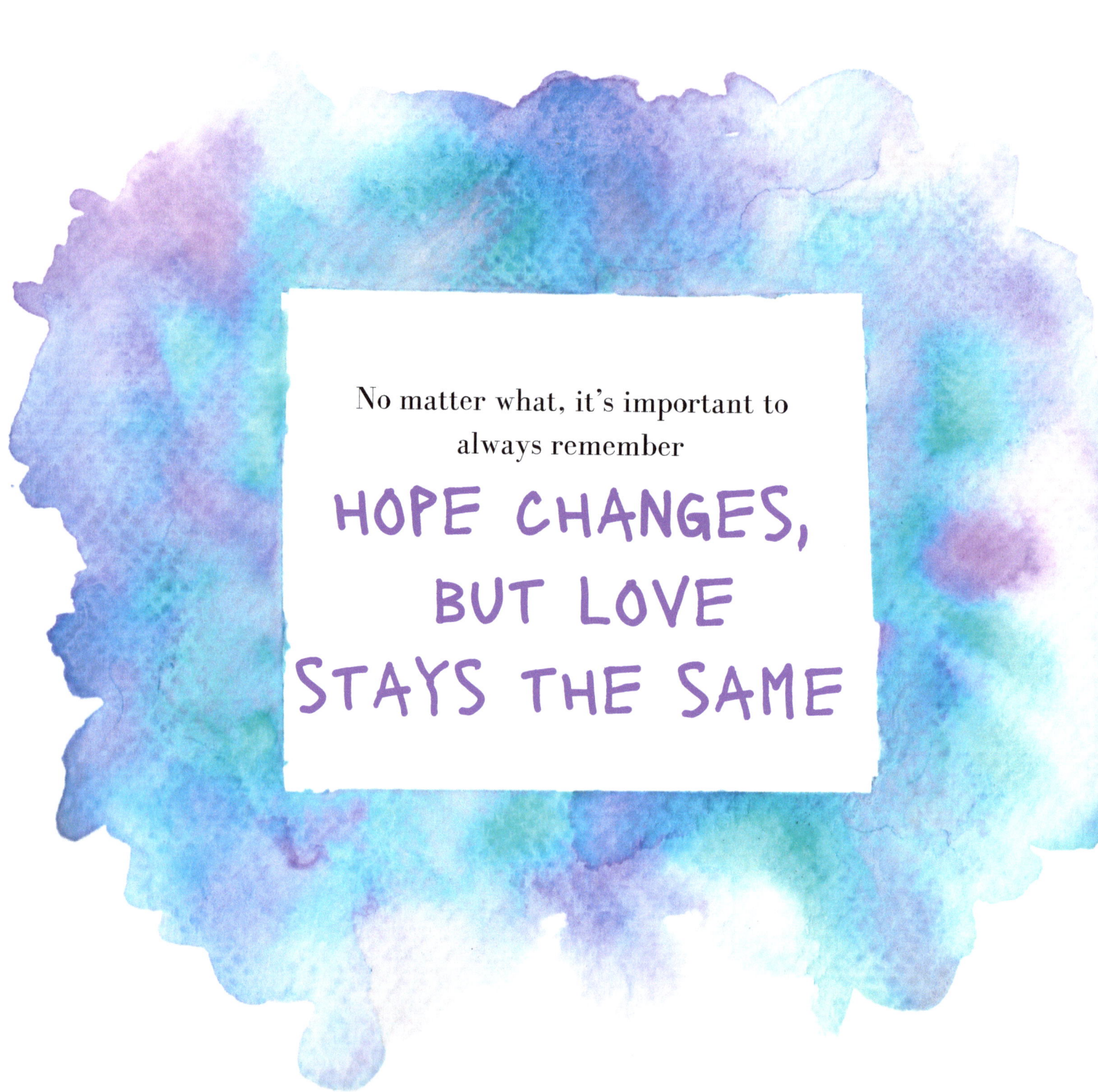

No matter what, it's important to always remember

HOPE CHANGES, BUT LOVE STAYS THE SAME

INFORMATION FOR GROWNUPS INDEX

MEDICAL EXPLANATIONS FOR KIDS

When explaining medical terms, diagnoses, or complications to kids, it is always best to keep it simple. Allow them to guide the conversation with questions, be as honest as possible, and don't be afraid to say, "I don't know, but we can ask and find out together."

If you aren't sure which organ system is most affected by your loved one's specific diagnosis, don't be afraid to ask your medical team. Sometimes diagnoses can affect different organ systems, so again, when explaining to kids, pick one or two at most to keep it simple for the initial conversation. You can explain more as time goes on if they are curious. Remember to follow their lead, and allow this to be a dynamic rather than a one-time conversation.

Child Life Specialists, social workers, or other psychosocial staff on your medical team may be able to help if you don't feel like your loved one's disease is captured in this short list and you need help explaining the illness or condition in a developmentally appropriate way.

Example from page 8: "As you may know, our person's body has been very sick. This is because they have brain cancer and now their brain is having trouble working like it is supposed to. This is a problem because their brain's job is to direct everything their body does like breathe, move, and think."

Here are some simple ways to explain what different body parts/organs do:

Heart: The heart's job is to pump blood through our body, which brings oxygen to all of our organs.

Blood/Circulatory System: The blood's job is to bring oxygen and nutrients to our organs so they can keep working.

Lungs: The lungs have the job of helping us breathe which helps get oxygen to our organs and brain.

Brain: The brain's job is to direct everything that happens in our body from moving and thinking and even things we don't know we are doing like breathing and our heart beating.

Kidneys/Urinary Tract: The kidneys are a filter for blood that keeps what our body needs and gets rid of things it doesn't need.

Liver: The liver cleans poisons out of our blood. It also helps make substances that our body needs.

Stomach/Gastrointestinal System: The stomach and intestines help digest our food and take out nutrients needed for the body to work and grow. It also gets rid of waste not needed by our body.

PREPARING YOUR CHILD

Setting the stage

Including your child in spending time with a dying loved one is a personal decision. If you feel like this is important to you and your family, it is helpful to prepare the child as much as possible with photos so they know what to expect, and also describe to them what they might hear, touch, smell, or feel in the room. The more sensory information you can provide, the more prepared a child will feel, and the less scary an unfamiliar situation will be.

Explaining equipment and machines

If your loved one has equipment such as breathing tubes, feeding tubes, IVs, or other equipment, you can explain what each of these machines does in simple terms: For example, an IV gives a person special medicine directly in their body, and a feeding tube brings food directly to their belly.

Explaining compassionate extubation/removal of mechanical support

If you are making the decision to remove mechanical support from your loved one in order to allow natural death, finding a way to explain this to a child can feel difficult. One way that might be helpful is: the machines are no longer helping our person's body, and their body is becoming very tired and uncomfortable. Even with the machine's help, their body is dying. We are going to remove the machines so they can be more comfortable. When we do that, we can hug and snuggle our person and tell them how much we love them. Without the machine's help, their body will stop working and they will die.

Explaining cancer

There is no one right way to explain cancer. When families have asked me, I have recommended explaining like this: Our body is made up of tiny things called cells. Cancer causes some cells to grow too fast and can hurt the body. Sometimes it causes bad cells to form in lumps called tumors which can stop the body from working like it should.

Seeing a loved one who has died

If your loved one has died and you want your child to see the body and say goodbye, you can explain that your person's body isn't working anymore and they have died. You can tell them that they can still touch their person if they choose, and you can explain that the body will feel cooler and may look paler than our bodies. Again, it is sometimes helpful to show children photos ahead of time. Allow your child to take the lead in this interaction. You can give them permission to interact with their person if they choose, and allow them to leave with a trusted adult if necessary. It can sometimes be helpful to identify a grown-up ahead of time who can take them out to the lobby/play room/car and spend time with them in the event your child needs to leave. This allows for you to spend precious time with your loved one and family, while also respecting your child's boundaries and feelings.

SUPPORTING YOUR CHILD & FAMILY

An important reminder

Please remember that there is no right or wrong way to have this conversation with kids. You are attempting to explain something that we, as adults, can have trouble explaining or understanding. Navigating the challenges of a terminal disease is challenging as an adult, let alone being tasked with explaining this to young minds.

When and how to revisit the conversation

It can feel difficult to find the "right time" to ask follow-up questions after initially sharing the news about your loved one's prognosis or reading this book together, but one way to check in frequently is to ask before an appointment: "Daddy/grandma/name has an appointment today. Do you have any questions you want to ask the doctor or nurse?" Another way to probe conversation is to be honest about how you're feeling. If your child catches you in a tearful or emotional moment and asks you what's wrong; instead of the knee-jerk: "I'm fine!," honestly answering the question can be helpful in modeling how to express difficult emotions in a healthy way.

How children understand death

Remember that children's understanding of death is much different than ours. Depending on their age, death is a very abstract concept, and will likely be better understood as years go on. Children are also naturally curious about death, and may ask lots of questions, sometimes repetitively. Do your best to keep your responses simple, clear, and consistent.

Importance of language

I generally recommend use concrete language like "death" and "dying," even if it feels hard to you. We, as grown-ups, prefer using terms like "pass away" or "transition" because it feels softer to us. To kids, it can be confusing because those terms don't hold the same meaning to them. I also recommend sharing the diagnosis name, as it can prevent generalizing the severity of the prognosis to any other sickness they encounter. For example, if they or someone else they care about catches the flu or a cold and you say they are sick, they may be less likely to become as afraid if they understand that a cold is not the same as cancer or whatever severe illness or injury their loved one has or had.

Who to ask for more help

If you have access to your medical team's psychosocial staff like social workers, Child Life Specialists or chaplains, feel free to include them and ask for their help with explaining your loved one's care and situation. It may not be easy, but if it is important to you and your family, they can help you.

Allowing appropriate choice

When we feel out of control, having the ability to make choices can feel empowering. Kids are no different in this. If you have the opportunity to decide where you or your loved one will die (e.g. at home or in the hospital), I encourage you to avoid making an assumption about what your child would feel comfortable with. Kids are adaptable and resilient and as long as they are prepared appropriately based on their developmental level, it's okay to allow them to decide how much they'd like to interact with their loved one. Just remember: with kids, open ended choice can feel overwhelming. Allowing them to choose between 2-3 choices (any of which you are also comfortable with) can allow them to feel empowered. This can also apply to funeral participation and attendance. Attending and participating in a funeral or memorial ritual can be very healing, especially with adequate preparation ahead of time.

A note about hope

Lastly, and I think most importantly: it is okay to maintain hope throughout this journey. Hope for healing, hope for a miracle, hope for effective treatment, hope for comfort, hope for time. Whatever this looks like to you, hold fast to your hope and don't let it go.

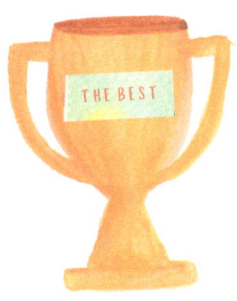

THE BEST

Thank you to my family for your
unending support and
encouragement

Thank you to Ami, Anne, Amanda,
and Brittney for your time, keen
eyes, passion, and expertise

My gratitude runs deep for you all.

ABOUT THE AUTHOR

Abigail Gellene-Beaudoin is a Licensed Clinical Social Worker (LCSW), Registered Play Therapist (RPT), and is certified in perinatal mental health (PMH-C). For nearly a decade, she dedicated her days to bringing comfort and joy to kids and families as a social worker in a pediatric and perinatal palliative care setting. Now, Abigail continues her journey of healing as a psychotherapist and play therapist at a counseling practice in Tidewater, Virginia, where she is dedicated to promoting resilience and hope, and fostering healing and connection amidst adversity.